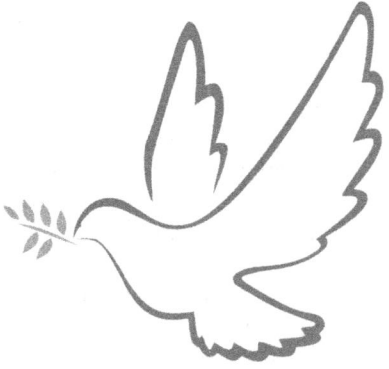

Suicide Hope Beyond A Moment

2025 © Janet Olivares
Published by Glorybound Publishing, Camp Verde, AZ
SAN 256-4564
Published in the United States of America
ISBN 9781607893738 1-60789-373-8
Copyright data is available on file.
Olivares, Janet, 1955-
  Suicide Hope Beyond A Moment /Janet Olivares
    Includes biographical reference.
1. Self-Help   2. Bible Books
I. Title

www.raphaccc.org
www.gloryboundpublishing.com

All rights reserved. No part of this publication may be reproduced, distributed, or transmitted in any form or by any means, including photocopying, recording or other electronic or mechanical methods without the prior written permission of the author, except in the case of brief quotations embodied in critical reviews and certain other non-commercial uses permitted by copyright laws.

Understand this book is not intended as a substitute for consultation with a licensed practitioner. Please consult with your own physician or health care specialist regarding the suggestions and/or recommendations in this book. The use of this book implies your acceptance of this disclaimer. Thank you.

Scripture quotations taken from the Holy Bible, New International Version®, NIV®. Copyright © 1973, 1978, 1984, 2011 by Biblica, Inc.™ Used by permission of Zondervan. All rights reserved worldwide.

For permissions, contact:
Rapha Christian Counseling Center & Academic Institute
1300 E Shaw, Suite 154
Fresno, CA 93710
www.raphaccc.org | info@raphaccc.org

Suicide
Hope Beyond a Moment

by Dr. Janet Olivares

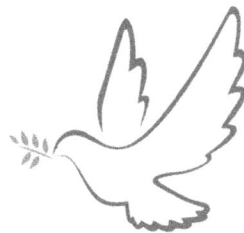

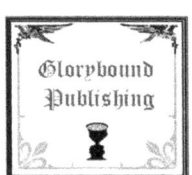

Glorybound Publishing
Camp Verde, Arizona USA
in the year 2025

Dedication

To the one who is fighting a battle no one can see
—this book is for you.

To every soul who has stared into the quiet and wondered if life still holds meaning,
may these pages whisper that you are seen, needed, and loved.

To the friend who listens, the counselor who stays late,
the pastor who prays, and the stranger who reaches out
—you are the hands of God in motion.

May this book be a reminder that darkness is not the end,
and that hope, once lit, can never be fully extinguished.
There is always another sunrise,
and God is still holding your right hand.

Foreword

There are moments in life that stop us in our tracks. Moments when words fail, faith trembles, and silence feels safer than speaking. For many, suicide is one of those moments — not because we do not care, but because we do not know what to say.

For years as a counselor, I have sat across from people who whispered what they thought no one would understand. They weren't trying to die — they were trying to stop the pain. They were searching for peace, for one voice that would remind them they were not alone.

This book was born from those sacred conversations. It is written for the one who is hurting and for the one who longs to help. It is for the mother who prays through tears, the pastor who carries quiet burdens, and the friend who fears saying the wrong thing. It is for every person who has ever wondered, "Where is God when despair feels louder than hope?"

The answer is: He is here. He has always been here.

Suicide is not the end of the story — it is a moment of thought, not an identity. And within that moment, God still reaches out His hand. He is the God who whispers, *"Do not fear; I will help you."* (Isaiah 41:13)

My prayer is that these pages will give you language for pain, courage for compassion, and faith for the journey toward healing. May you discover that hope is not gone — it is waiting in the very space where you thought it had died. If you are reading this and feel the weight of despair, please pause. Reach for help. Call or text **988** for the Suicide and Crisis Lifeline. You are not alone. God is not finished with your story.

To every counselor, pastor, parent, and friend — may you be reminded that one word, one presence, one prayer can save a life. You are the bridge between the moment of thought and the miracle of hope.

Heavenly Father,
May this book be light in dark places. May every reader feel Your nearness and know that Your love never fails. Teach us to see others the way You see them — worthy, loved, and held. Amen.

Table of Contents

Introduction – Suicide – Hope Beyond the Moment...10

Chapter 1: What Suicide Is — and What It Isn't... 19
Chapter 2: The Science of a Moment... 23
Chapter 3: Risk Factors and Warning Signs... 28
Chapter 4: Faith, Despair, and Hope... 33
Chapter 5: Immediate Steps in Crisis...38
Chapter 6: Treatment and Healing Pathways... 43
Chapter 7: Stories of Turning Points... 48
Chapter 8: Families, Friends, and Pastors... 52
Chapter 9: The Church as a Lifeline... 57
Chapter 10: After a Crisis — Healing the Soul... 60
Chapter 11: Grief and the Aftermath...67
Chapter 12: Prevention at Scale...72
Conclusion: Life Beyond the Moment...77

Letters of Hope and Healing: God Is Still Holding Your Hand...71

Appendices
Appendix A: Personal Safety Plan...90
Appendix B: Conversation Scripts...92
Appendix C: Scriptures of Hope...95
Appendix D: Resources...96

About the Author...98

Introduction

Suicide. It is one of the heaviest words in our language. For some, it carries the ache of losing a loved one. For others, it is a word they whisper in shame, attached to thoughts they wish they never had. And for far too many, it is a word they never got the chance to speak aloud before it claimed their life.

This book begins with a conviction that may sound startling: suicide is a moment of thought, not a mental illness.

Why make such a claim? Because too often suicide has been framed as a permanent mark on a person's identity — as if it means they are defined by mental illness, beyond hope or change. Yet the truth is far more complex, and far more hopeful. Suicidal ideation can come in a sudden, overwhelming moment — a collapse of perspective where the mind becomes convinced that no way forward exists. And yet, just as quickly as such thoughts arrive, they can pass. When a person survives the moment, life continues. Healing, faith, and hope remain possible.

A Thought, Not an Identity

To say suicide is a "moment of thought" does not mean it is small or unimportant. On the contrary, it is deadly serious. But it reframes suicide in a way that brings freedom and hope: a thought is not who you are.

Mental illness can certainly increase vulnerability. Depression, anxiety, trauma, and other diagnoses are well-documented risk factors. But suicide itself is not a diagnosis. Not every person with a mental illness contemplates suicide, and not every person who has suicidal thoughts carries a diagnosis.

When we treat suicide only as a "mental illness," we risk turning a temporary crisis into a permanent identity. That is not only untrue — it is dangerous. What we believe about suicide shapes how we respond to it. If we believe it is unchangeable, we lose urgency for intervention. But if we see it as a thought — as a moment that can pass — we are more likely to respond with compassion, immediacy, and hope.

The Narrow Hallway of Despair

Suicidal thinking often feels like walking down a hallway where all the doors are shut. The mind whispers: there is no way out. This "tunnel vision" is a well-studied phenomenon — a crisis of perception where options seem to vanish.

But here is the truth: there are doors. They may not be visible in the moment, but they exist. Hope, help, community, faith, and healing are doors that can open when someone is not left alone in despair. The hallway of suicidal thought is real, but it is not endless.

The Role of Faith

For those of us who hold to faith in Christ, suicide is not only a social and medical concern but a spiritual one. Scripture reminds us:

"The Lord is close to the brokenhearted and saves those who are crushed in spirit." (Psalm 34:18)

God does not condemn those in despair. He draws near. Jesus Himself, in Gethsemane, confessed to being "overwhelmed with sorrow to the point of death" (Matthew 26:38). Despair is not foreign to our Savior. This means those who struggle with suicidal thoughts are not beyond His reach; they are precisely the ones He came to comfort.

Faith offers more than comfort. It offers meaning, forgiveness, and the assurance that our worth is not determined by our darkest thoughts. We are made in God's image, and no moment of despair can erase that truth.

Why This Book?

I wrote this book because too many lives are being lost — not because people are permanently broken, but because they believed a lie in a moment of pain. They believed the lie that there was no hope. They believed the lie that their life had no worth. They believed that the thought was final.

This book is here to declare: the thought is not final. The crisis can be survived. Life can be lived.

I also wrote this for families, pastors, counselors, and friends who long to help but feel helpless. You will find practical tools here: how to recognize warning signs, what to say in a crisis, how to walk with someone after the moment has passed, and how to create communities that bring light into darkness.

What You Will Find in These Pages

This book is structured in three parts:

1. **Understanding the Moment**
   We will explore what suicide is — and what it is not. You will learn the difference between a moment of thought and a lifelong identity, how the brain and body react in crisis, and why seeing suicide as a "moment" change everything.

2. **Responding to the Moment**
   Here we will discuss practical steps for crisis response: what to do when someone is at risk, how to talk about suicide without shame, and how to create safety in the most urgent hours.

3. **Living Beyond the Moment**
   The final section will focus on recovery, prevention, and hope. We will look at how faith, community, and purpose empower people to not only survive suicidal thoughts but to thrive beyond them. We will also discuss how churches and communities can be lifelines of support.

At the end of the book, you will find appendices with safety planning tools, sample conversation guides, and national/international crisis resources.

A Word of Safety

Before we continue, I must say this clearly: if you are in crisis right now, do not wait to finish this book. Please, pause and reach for help immediately. If you are in the United States, dial or text **988** for the Suicide & Crisis Lifeline. If you are outside the U.S., look for your local crisis hot-line or emergency number. This book is meant to guide and encourage, but your life is too valuable to wait for the next page.

Final Word of Introduction

My heart is to remove shame, break stigma, and offer hope. Suicide is not a verdict. It is not destiny. It is not a life sentence.

It is a moment of thought.
And with God's help, with compassionate people, and with practical tools, that moment can pass — leaving life, purpose, and hope in it's wake.

Chapter 1: What Suicide Is — and What It Isn't

- Clarify definitions: suicidal ideation, suicide attempt, death by suicide.
- Debunk myths e.g., "talking about suicide makes it worse."
- Contrast "moment of thought" vs. "lifelong identity."
- Emphasize hope: thoughts are real but not final.

Chapter 2: The Science of a Moment

- How stress, trauma, and biology narrow thinking "tunnel vision."
- The role of the brain in crisis: amygdala hijack, cortisol.
- Why moments feel permanent even though they are not.
- Practical takeaway: moments pass — intervention buys life.

Chapter 3: Risk Factors and Warning Signs

- Mental health conditions: depression, PTSD, substance use.
- Life stressors: loss, isolation, shame, financial strain.
- Immediate warning signs with checklist.
- The power of noticing: how awareness prevents tragedy.

Chapter 4: Faith, Despair, and Hope

- Biblical examples of despair: Elijah, David, Job, Jesus in Gethsemane.
- God's nearness to the brokenhearted Psalm 34:18.
- How faith provides worth, identity, and purpose.
- Addressing stigma in the church.

Chapter 5: Immediate Steps in Crisis

- Five practical steps for helpers: stay, ask, remove means, call, follow-up.
- Sample questions & scripts for talking with someone at risk.
- Safety planning basics.
- Callout boxes: 988 (U.S.), international lifelines.

Chapter 6: Treatment and Healing Pathways

- Overview of counseling, therapy, medication, support groups.
- The difference between treating illness and supporting crisis.
- Integration of faith and evidence-based care.
- Importance of follow-up after hospitalization or crisis intervention.

Chapter 7: Stories of Turning Points

- Vignettes of people who survived suicidal thoughts.
- Focus on what helped them: support, faith, intervention.
- Hopeful outcomes: life beyond the moment.
- Callout reflection questions for readers.

Chapter 8: Families, Friends, and Pastors

- The role of loved ones: what to say, what not to say.
- Boundaries for helpers (don't carry it alone).
- Pastoral care: being present without judgment.
- Community follow-up and long-term support.

Chapter 9: The Church as a Lifeline

- Creating safe spaces where people can admit suicidal thoughts.
- Training pastors and leaders to respond wisely.
- Developing small-group support and prayer teams.
- Church partnerships with mental health professionals.

Chapter 10: After a Crisis — Healing the Soul

- Recovery after a suicide attempt.
- Dealing with shame, guilt, or spiritual questions.
- Practices of hope: prayer, gratitude, community, serving others.
- Rebuilding identity and purpose.

Chapter 11: Grief and the Aftermath

- For families who have lost someone.
- Processing grief with honesty and faith.
- Avoiding blame.
- How God meets us in loss.

Chapter 12: Prevention at Scale

- Public health: means restriction, training (QPR, ASIST).
- Policy efforts and school-based prevention.
- Global perspective (WHO, CDC).
- Why every life matters to the community.

Conclusion: Life Beyond the Moment

- Reaffirm the central message: suicide is a thought, not an identity.
- Hope and worth in Christ.
- Call to action: speak openly, respond quickly, build communities of care.

Appendices

A. Safety Plan Template (fillable).

B. Conversation Scripts "How to ask if someone is suicidal."

C. Scripture Promises of Hope for daily meditation.

D. Resource List: U.S. 988 Lifeline, international hotlines, AFSP, WHO.

Chapter 1
– What Suicide Is — and What It Isn't–

Suicide is one of the most misunderstood subjects in our culture and even within the church. For too long, it has been spoken about in hushed tones, covered with shame, or avoided altogether. Misunderstanding leads to stigma, and stigma prevents people from reaching for help. To begin this journey, we must first be clear about what suicide truly is—and what it is not.

Suicide Is Real, But It Is Not an Identity

When a person experiences suicidal thoughts, they often feel as though those thoughts define them. They may think, "If I am having these thoughts, I must be hopeless. I must be broken. I must be my illness." But suicidal ideation is not an identity. It does not mean someone is permanently defective.

Suicide is, at it's core, a moment of thought—a crisis of perception and emotion. It is an intersection of pain, hopelessness, and often exhaustion. It is real, it is serious, but it is not permanent. Thoughts can shift. Feelings can change. Life can continue beyond the moment.

Suicide Is Not Always About Mental Illness

One of the most common misconceptions is that only people with "mental illness" experience suicidal thoughts. While conditions like depression, PTSD, or bipolar disorder may increase risk, not everyone who has suicidal thoughts carries a diagnosis. And not everyone with a diagnosis contemplates suicide.

Suicide is far more complex. It can be triggered by loss, financial strain, family conflict, trauma, shame, or spiritual despair. To reduce suicide only to "mental illness" is to miss the larger picture—and to risk making people believe they are locked into an identity they cannot escape.

Suicide Is Not Selfishness

Another harmful myth is that suicide is an act of selfishness. This is deeply untrue. People in suicidal crisis are not thinking of themselves first; they are often convinced wrongly that their death would relieve a burden on others. The thought process is distorted, not malicious. To call someone selfish for their despair only deepens shame and pushes them further into silence.

Suicide Is Not Unforgivable

For centuries, the church has sometimes treated suicide as an unforgivable sin. But Scripture reminds us that nothing can separate us from the love of God in Christ Jesus (Romans 8:38–39). Despair does not erase grace. Jesus met people in their lowest moments, including Elijah under the broom tree who prayed, "I have had enough, Lord. Take my life." (1 Kings 19:4). God did not condemn Elijah. He fed him, gave him rest, and restored him for his journey.

When the church understands that despair is not damnation, it can become a refuge rather than a place of silence and shame.

Suicide Is a Moment of Thought

This is the central conviction of this book: suicide is a moment of thought, not a lifelong sentence. For some, the thought may be brief, fleeting, and pass without action. For others, it may return repeatedly during times of stress or pain. But in every case, the thought itself is not destiny.

Why does this matter? Because if suicide is seen as a permanent identity, people may feel they are beyond help. But if it is seen as a moment of thought serious, but temporarily help becomes possible, and hope becomes real.

Suicide Can Be Prevented

Research and experience both show that suicide is preventable. Intervention works. Crisis lines save lives. Supportive presence changes outcomes. When someone is kept safe through the moment, they can go on to live full, meaningful lives.

Every conversation matters. Every safe presence matters. Every prayer matters.

▶ Reflection

- What assumptions have I made about suicide?
- How have those beliefs shaped the way I talk—or avoid talking about it?
- How might seeing suicide as a "moment of thought" change the way I respond to others and to myself.

♥ Scripture for Hope

"The Lord is close to the brokenhearted and saves those who are crushed in spirit." (Psalm 34:18)

"For I know the plans I have for you," declares the Lord, "plans to prosper you and not to harm you, plans to give you hope and a future." (Jeremiah 29:11)

Reflections and Prayer

Chapter 2
– The Science of a Moment –

When people think of suicide, they often imagine it as the slow collapse of a life, a long decline with no turning point. But for many, suicidal ideation emerges in an instant an acute crisis when pain outweighs perspective. This chapter explores what happens in the human brain and body during that moment, why it feels so overwhelming, and how understanding both science and faith reveals hope beyond despair.

The Brain in Crisis

Our brains are God's intricate design, but under stress they can shift into survival mode. When the amygdala — the brain's alarm system senses threat, it floods the body with stress hormones like adrenaline and cortisol. This response is useful when escaping physical danger, but during emotional pain it can hijack the ability to think clearly.

When the prefrontal cortex (the logical part of the brain) goes offline, perspective narrows. Instead of seeing multiple solutions, the brain clings to the one that seems to end the pain fastest. In that fragile state, suicide may appear as the only door out.

Survivor Story: "I Just Wanted the Pain to Stop"

"It wasn't that I wanted to die. I just wanted the pain to stop. My mind kept telling me, 'there's no other way.' Looking back, it's strange because I had people who cared and options I didn't see. But in that moment, I felt blind to all of it."
— Anonymous survivor

This story echoes what many who survive suicide attempts later say: the desire wasn't truly for death, but for relief. Their crisis brain made relief and death feel synonymous but only in that moment.

Tunnel Vision and Cognitive Narrowing

Psychologists call this cognitive narrowing tunnel vision of the mind. When someone is in suicidal crisis, options vanish from awareness. Hope disappears. A hallway with many doors becomes a hallway with none.

Outside of crisis, that same person can see options clearly: therapy, prayer, community, new opportunities. But inside the moment, the brain blocks them out. This explains why survivors often reflect: "I don't know what I was thinking. I just couldn't see any other way."

The Role of Exhaustion and Overload

Suicidal crises rarely come from one cause. Instead, they build through layers of pressure:

- Emotional burdens: grief, rejection, shame.
- Physical strain: chronic illness, pain, or sheer exhaustion.
- Environmental factors: financial collapse, family conflict, isolation.
- Substance use: alcohol and drugs can intensify impulsivity.

Each layer is like weight on a scale. When the final ounce is added, the balance tips into crisis. That tipping point often surprises the person themselves: "I didn't think it would hit me like that."

Survivor Story: "It Felt Like a Switch Flipped"

"I had been under stress for months, but I was still pushing through. Then one night after an argument, it was like a switch flipped in my head. Suddenly, all I could think was, end it.' The thought was so fast, so forceful. But later, I couldn't believe I came that close. It really was a moment."

Why the Moment Passes

The encouraging truth is that suicidal crises are often short-lived. Research shows the most intense urge typically lasts minutes to hours. If safety and support are present, the wave passes.

This is why crisis lines, prayer partners, and compassionate listeners save lives. They keep a person safe long enough for the moment to fade and perspective to return.

Sidebar: Brain Science in Plain Language

- Amygdala: Alarm bell of the brain. Helpful for physical danger, but can overreact in emotional pain.
- Prefrontal cortex: The "logic" center. It goes quiet in crisis, making decisions feel urgent and distorted.
- Cortisol: Stress hormone that increases tunnel vision.
- Good news: Once the stress response calms, the thinking brain re-engages, and hope reappears.

Practical Tools to Calm the Brain

When someone feels trapped in crisis, small steps can help deactivate the alarm system:

1. Breathing prayer: Inhale slowly: "Be still." Exhale: "And know that I am God." (Psalm 46:10)
2. Grounding exercise: Name five things you see, four you feel, three you hear, two you smell, one you taste. This pulls the brain out of tunnel vision.
3. Movement: A short walk, a splash of cold water, or stretching can break the cycle of panic.
4. Call a lifeline: In the U.S., dial or text 988 for immediate support. Outside the U.S., use your local crisis hot-line.

These tools don't solve every problem, but they buy time — and in suicide prevention, time saves lives.

Faith Meets Science

The Bible is honest about despair. Even Paul confessed:

"We were under great pressure, far beyond our ability to endure, so that we despaired of life itself... But this happened that we might not rely on ourselves but on God, who raises the dead." (2 Corinthians 1:8–9)

Despair did not end Paul's story. God carried him beyond the moment. Science affirms what faith declares: crisis is real but temporary, and hope is possible.

▶ Reflection

- Have I ever felt tunnel vision in stress, where options seemed invisible?
- What tools can I use to calm my body and mind when overwhelmed?
- How does knowing that suicidal urges are short-lived change the way I view them?

♥ Scripture for Hope

"Even though I walk through the darkest valley, I will fear no evil, for you are with me; your rod and your staff, they comfort me." (Psalm 23:4)

Reflections and Prayer

Chapter 3
– Risk Factors and Warning Signs –

Suicide rarely happens without warning. While the final moment may appear suddenly, there are often patterns, signals, and risk factors that build over time. By learning to recognize them, we can step into someone's life before the crisis becomes overwhelming. Awareness is not about fear it is about hope. The more we understand the signs, the more prepared we are to help.

Understanding Risk Factors

Risk factors are the underlying conditions or experiences that increase the likelihood someone may consider suicide. They do not guarantee a person will become suicidal, but they increase vulnerability.

Some of the most common include:

- Mental health challenges: depression, PTSD, bipolar disorder, anxiety, and substance use.
- Past trauma: abuse, violence, or unresolved grief.
- Chronic stress: financial struggles, job loss, relationship breakdowns.
- Isolation: lack of social support, feeling unwanted or alone.
- Chronic pain or illness: physical suffering that erodes hope.
- History of suicide attempts: prior crises increase risk of future attempts.

Each factor alone may not lead to suicidal thoughts. But together, they can create a heavy burden one that feels unbearable without help.

Protective Factors: What Pushes Back

Just as risk factors increase vulnerability, protective factors reduce it. These are strengths, supports, and resources that give people reasons to live. Some include:

- Strong faith and belief in God's purpose.
- Supportive relationships with family, friends, and community.
- Access to mental health care and counseling.
- Skills for problem-solving and managing emotions.
- Involvement in meaningful work, service, or ministry.

Protective factors don't eliminate despair, but they provide anchors in the storm. They remind someone that life is worth holding onto.

Warning Signs in Daily Life

Risk factors are background conditions. Warning signs are what we see or hear in the present moment signals that someone may be thinking about suicide now. These include:

- Talking about wanting to die or feeling like a burden.
- Withdrawing from friends, family, or activities once enjoyed.
- Increased use of alcohol or drugs.
- Sudden mood swings — extreme sadness, then calm after deciding.
- Giving away prized possessions.
- Talking about hopelessness or having no reason to live.
- Searching online for methods or means.

The presence of warning signs does not mean someone will act, but it should always be taken seriously. It is far better to ask and be wrong than to stay silent and risk losing a life.

The Importance of Asking Directly

One of the strongest tools we have is asking the question plainly: "Are you thinking about suicide?" Many fear that speaking the word will "plant the idea." Research shows the opposite. Asking directly communicates care and can relieve the burden of secrecy.

When asked compassionately, people are often grateful. It tells them, "I see you. I care. You don't have to carry this alone

Faith and Risk Factors

The Bible is honest about despair. Elijah, Job, Jeremiah, and even Jesus experienced moments of deep anguish. Yet God's response was always presence, provision, and hope.

"Cast all your anxiety on Him because He cares for you." (1 Peter 5:7)

Risk factors remind us of human weakness. Scripture reminds us of divine strength. Both are real. Both must be acknowledged. And together they show us the need for both practical help and spiritual hope.

Survivor Story: "The Signs Were There"

"Looking back, I realize I was dropping hints all the time. I said things like, 'I'm tired of living this way,' or 'you'd be better off without me.' I started skipping church and stopped answering calls. At the time, I hoped someone would notice, but I didn't know how to ask for help."

Stories like this remind us that warning signs are often subtle but they are present. Our attentiveness may save a life.

What Families, Friends, and Churches Can Do

- Pay attention to changes in mood, speech, or behavior.
- Ask directly if you are concerned.
- Listen without judgment. Do not argue, minimize, or try to "fix."
- Offer connection to professional help and crisis resources.
- Stay present. Sometimes the most powerful act is simply not leaving someone alone.

Churches can play a vital role by teaching leaders to recognize risk factors, creating safe spaces for honest conversations, and reminding people that they are not defined by their darkest thoughts.

▶ Reflection

- Which of these risk factors or warning signs have I seen in myself or others?
- How might I respond differently the next time I notice them?
- What protective factors can I strengthen in my own life right now?

♥ Scripture for Hope

"The Lord is my strength and my shield; my heart trusts in Him, and He helps me." (Psalm 28:7)

Reflections and Prayer

Chapter 4
– Faith, Despair, and Hope –

Suicidal thoughts are not only psychological or emotional; they are deeply spiritual. Scripture shows us that even the most faithful servants of God experienced crushing despair. Yet in every story, we also see God's nearness, compassion, and restoration. Understanding despair through the lens of faith allows us to see that hopelessness is never the end of the story.

Biblical Voices of Despair

The Bible does not shy away from human anguish:

- Elijah sat under the broom tree and prayed, "I have had enough, Lord. Take my life." (1 Kings 19:4)

- Job cursed the day of his birth, overwhelmed by suffering (Job 3:1–11).

- Jeremiah cried out, "Why did I ever come out of the womb to see trouble and sorrow?" (Jeremiah 20:18).

- Jesus Himself, in Gethsemane, said, "My soul is overwhelmed with sorrow to the point of death." (Matthew 26:38).

These examples reveal a vital truth: despair is not a sign of weak faith. It is part of the human condition. God's people have always wrestled with moments of hopelessness

God's Response to Despair

When Elijah asked for death, God did not scold him. Instead, He sent an angel with food and rest (1 Kings 19:5–7). God's first response was compassion, not condemnation.

This is God's heart toward all who despair: presence, provision, and restoration. He is "close to the brokenhearted and saves those who are crushed in spirit" (Psalm 34:18). He draws near in our darkest valleys.

The Lie of Hopelessness

Despair often whispers the lie: "There is no future. There is no way out." But Scripture confronts that lie with truth:

"For I know the plans I have for you," declares the Lord, "plans to prosper you and not to harm you, plans to give you hope and a future." (Jeremiah 29:11)

Hopelessness tells us the story is over. God tells us He is still writing.

Faith as a Protective Factor

Research shows that faith and spirituality can reduce suicide risk by giving people meaning, community, and a sense of purpose. But beyond the statistics, faith reminds us that our worth does not rest on how we feel. It rests on who God says we are: His beloved children.

Faith provides:

- Identity: We are made in God's image (Genesis 1:27).
- Purpose: Our lives are part of His plan (Ephesians 2:10).
- Community: The body of Christ carries one another's burdens (Galatians 6:2).
- Hope: Christ overcame death itself (1 Corinthians 15:55–57).

When Faith Communities Cause Harm

Sadly, not all churches have responded well to despair. Some have labeled it as weakness or sin, leaving people feeling shame rather than supported. This must change. The church should be the safest place to speak openly about pain. Judgment silences, but compassion free.

Survivor Story: "The Church That Listened"

"When I told my pastor I was thinking about ending my life, I expected him to quote verses and tell me to 'just have more faith.' Instead, he sat with me and cried. He prayed with me, but he also helped me call a counselor. That moment saved me. It showed me that God cared enough to put someone in my path who listened."

This is the kind of faith-filled response that heals: listening, praying, and guiding toward practical help.

Hope in Christ

Christian hope is not naïve optimism. It is rooted in the resurrection of Jesus, who conquered death itself. Because Christ lives, despair never has the final word.

"Praise be to the God and Father of our Lord Jesus Christ! In His great mercy He has given us new birth into a living hope through the resurrection of Jesus Christ from the dead." (1 Peter 1:3)

This hope is "living" it is active, enduring, and stronger than the darkest thoughts.

Practical Ways Faith Can Help

- Scripture meditation: Speaking God's promises aloud when lies of despair arise.
- Prayer practices: Honest prayers of lament, as seen in the Psalms.
- Worship: Singing truths that lift the heart above present pain.
- Community: Small groups, prayer partners, and accountability.
- Service: Helping others reminds us of our purpose and worth.

▶ Reflection

- How have I seen despair in the lives of biblical figures or in my own life?
- What lies have despair whispered to me, and what truths from Scripture counter them?
- How can my church become a refuge for those who feel hopeless?

♥ Scripture for Hope

"The Lord is my shepherd, I lack nothing. He makes me lie down in green pastures, He leads me beside quiet waters, He refreshes my soul." (Psalm 23:1–3)

-

Reflections and Prayer

Chapter 5
– Immediate Steps in Crisis –

A suicidal crisis can feel overwhelming for everyone involved both the person in despair and the loved one trying to help. Yet hope lies in knowing there are clear, simple steps we can take in the moment. These actions do not require special training; they require compassion, presence, and the willingness to stay.

Step 1: Stay Present

The first and most powerful response is to simply stay. Do not leave the person alone if they are in immediate danger. Your presence communicates: "You matter. You are not alone in this."

- Sit nearby, even in silence.
- Offer calm reassurance: "I'm here with you."
- Eliminate distractions and give full attention.

Presence is a lifeline. Many people survive a suicidal crisis because someone refuses to walk away.

Step 2: Ask Directly

It can feel frightening to ask the question, but research shows it is lifesaving. Use clear, compassionate language:

- "Are you thinking about suicide?"
- "Have you thought about hurting yourself?"

Avoid vague questions like "You're not thinking of doing something silly, are you?" Directness shows courage and communicates that it is safe to tell the truth.

Step 3: Remove Access to Means

If possible, gently ensure that dangerous items are out of reach. This could mean:

- Safely storing medications.
- Removing firearms from the home.
- Staying with the person until they are in a safer environment.

Reducing access to lethal means saves lives. Even small barriers can give enough time for the crisis to pass.

Step 4: Call for Help

No one should carry the weight of a suicidal crisis alone. Reach out immediately:

- In the U.S., dial or text 988 for the Suicide & Crisis Lifeline.
- If outside the U.S., find your local crisis number or call emergency services.
- Contact a trusted counselor, pastor, or family member who can provide ongoing support.

If the person is in imminent danger, do not hesitate to call 911 (or your local emergency number). Safety must come first.

Step 5: Follow Up

Crisis intervention does not end when the moment passes. Follow up with:

- A text or phone call the next day: "I'm thinking of you. How are you feeling now?"
- Offering to attend counseling or a doctor's appointment together.

- Encouraging participation in faith community or support groups.

Consistent follow-up reinforces that the person's life matters and that their presence is valued.

Sample Scripts for Helping Conversations

- "I can see you're in a lot of pain. I'm not going anywhere. Can you tell me what you're thinking?"
- "It sounds like you're feeling trapped. I want to help you find a way through this."
- "I care about you too much to let you carry this alone. Let's reach out together for more help."

Short, compassionate statements open the door for honesty and support.

Faith in the Crisis Moment

Prayer and Scripture can provide immediate comfort in the darkest hour. But remember timing and sensitivity matter. Sometimes silence and presence come first, followed by gentle prayer.

"God is our refuge and strength, an ever-present help in trouble." (Psalm 46:1)

When invited, pray aloud: "Lord, we feel overwhelmed right now. Bring peace, bring light, and remind us of Your presence."

What Not to Say

Avoid phrases that minimize or condemn:

- "You just need more faith."
- "You're being selfish."
- "Other people have it worse."

These responses increase shame. Instead, focus on empathy and truth: "You are loved. You are not alone. God is with you.

▶ Reflection

- How comfortable am I with asking directly about suicide?
- Who could I call right now if I needed support in helping someone?
- What can my church or family put in place to be ready for a crisis moment?

♥ Scripture for Hope

"When you pass through the waters, I will be with you; and when you pass through the rivers, they will not sweep over you." (Isaiah 43:2)

Reflections and Prayer

Chapter 6
– Treatment and Healing Pathways –

Surviving a suicidal crisis is only the beginning. Healing requires more than making it through one moment; it requires learning to live beyond despair, finding support, and restoring hope. Treatment and healing are not one-size-fits-all. They involve physical, emotional, relational, and spiritual dimensions. In this chapter, we will explore how practical care, professional support, and faith work together to create pathways of recovery.

Why Treatment Matters

Many people who experience suicidal thoughts never seek professional help. Fear, shame, and stigma often keep them silent. Yet untreated pain can linger and grow heavier over time. Treatment provides new tools, safe spaces, and ongoing support that can save lives and restore hope.

Seeking help is not weakness. It is courage. Proverbs reminds us:

"Plans fail for lack of counsel, but with many advisers they succeed." (Proverbs 15:22)

Just as we would see a doctor for a broken bone, we should seek help for emotional wounds.

Counseling and Therapy

Professional counseling is one of the most effective ways to address the pain behind suicidal thoughts. Counselors provide:

- Safe listening spaces without judgment.

- Tools for managing thoughts, emotions, and stress.
- Support for processing trauma, loss, or abuse.

Evidence-based therapies include:

- Cognitive Behavioral Therapy (CBT): Helps identify and challenge harmful thought patterns.
- Dialectical Behavior Therapy (DBT): Teaches skills for managing intense emotions and reducing self-harm.
- Trauma-informed counseling: Addresses wounds from past abuse, violence, or neglect.

Counseling is not only clinical, it can also integrate faith, prayer, and Scripture for holistic healing.

Medication and Medical Support

For some, biological factors contribute to depression and suicidal thinking. Medication prescribed by a doctor or psychiatrist can help rebalance the brain's chemistry. While medication is not a cure-all, it can be an important part of recovery.

Just as we accept insulin for diabetes or chemotherapy for cancer, there is no shame in receiving medical support for the brain. God often uses medicine as a means of healing

Community and Support Group

Healing rarely happens in isolation. Support groups — whether in churches, community centers, or online — provide encouragement and accountability. Sharing struggles with others who understand reduces shame and creates belonging.

- Faith-based groups remind participants of God's presence.
- Peer support groups offer understanding from those with lived experience.
- Family groups teach loved ones how to walk alongside with wisdom and compassion.

The Role of the Church in Healing

The church can be a bridge to healing when it embraces compassion and honesty. Practical ways churches can help include:

- Hosting support groups or prayer circles for those in despair.
- Training leaders to recognize warning signs and respond appropriately.
- Partnering with local counselors and crisis centers.
- Offering sermons and Bible studies that speak openly about hope, despair, and God's love.

When the church avoids the subject of suicide, silence becomes harmful. When the church speaks with truth and love, it becomes a refuge.

Faith as a Healing Pathway

Faith does not erase pain instantly, but it provides meaning and hope that treatment alone cannot supply. Healing in Christ includes:

- Identity: Knowing I am God's child, not my diagnosis.
- Hope: Believing my story is not finished.
- Peace: Receiving God's comfort through prayer and His Word.
- Strength: Trusting in His power when my own strength runs out.

"He heals the brokenhearted and binds up their wounds." (Psalm 147:3)

Survivor Story: "Counseling and Christ Together"

"When I first started counseling, I felt ashamed. I thought it meant I didn't trust God enough. But my counselor prayed with me and reminded me that God often heals through people. Over time, I realized that therapy and faith weren't in conflict they were working together. Christ was healing me through counseling.

Building a Long-Term Healing Plan

Healing is not instant. It is a process. A strong plan includes:

1. Professional care — counselor, therapist, or doctor.
2. Faith practices — prayer, Bible reading, worship.
3. Healthy rhythms — rest, exercise, nutrition.
4. Community — support from church, family, and friends.
5. Purpose — setting goals, serving others, rediscovering meaning.

Healing is possible when all these pieces work together.

▶ Reflection

- What barriers might keep me (or others) from seeking help?
- How can I view counseling and faith as partners rather than opposites?
- Who in my life could I walk with on their healing journey?

♥ Scripture for Hope

"Come to me, all you who are weary and burdened, and I will give you rest." (Matthew 11:28)

Reflections and Prayer

Chapter 7
– Stories of Turning Points –

Statistics can tell us the scope of suicide, but stories reveal the heart of it. Numbers show trends; stories show lives. In this chapter, we will listen to voices of those who faced suicidal thoughts and survived. Their testimonies remind us that the moment of despair does not have the final word. With support, faith, and courage, there is always a turning point.

Why Stories Matter

Survivor stories break stigma. They say to others: "You are not the only one." They also offer proof that suicidal thoughts are often temporary and that help can lead to healing. When told responsibly, these stories provide hope without glamorizing despair.

"Let the redeemed of the Lord tell their story those He redeemed from the hand of the foe." (Psalm 107:2)

Turning Point: A Pastor's Embrace

"I had decided it was over. That Sunday morning, I walked into church planning to say goodbye. My pastor stopped me at the door, looked me in the eye, and said, 'You matter more than you know.' He had no idea what I was planning, but that one sentence stopped me. I broke down, and for the first time, I asked for help."

This story reminds us that sometimes a single caring word can be a lifeline.

Turning Point: A Friend Who Stayed

"One night, I told my friend I was done. She didn't panic or lecture me. She just said, 'Then I'm staying with you tonight.' She sat on my floor, prayed with me, and made sure I wasn't alone. The next day, she helped me call a counselor. Looking back, that night was the difference between death and life."

Presence — simple, quiet, faithful often matters more than perfect words.

Turning Point: A Crisis Line Call

"At 2 a.m., I was sitting with a bottle of pills in my hand. For some reason, I remembered seeing a commercial about a hotline. I dialed. A calm voice answered, 'I'm glad you called. Tell me what's going on.' For the next hour, a stranger listened to my pain. By the end of the call, the urge had passed. That phone call saved me."

This story shows the power of crisis services. In the U.S., the number is 988. For those outside the U.S., national crisis lines offer similar support.

Faith as the Turning Point

"I had lost everything job, marriage, home. I sat in my car crying, asking God if there was any reason to go on. Suddenly, the verse came to mind: 'I will never leave you nor forsake you.' (Hebrews 13:5) It wasn't a loud voice, but a whisper in my spirit. That whisper gave me just enough strength to drive to my sister's house instead of giving up."

God often speaks into despair with reminders of His presence. Faith can be the lifeline that shifts a moment of hopelessness into a step toward life.

Common Threads in Turning Points

Across these stories, we see patterns:

- Someone noticed. A pastor, friend, or stranger reached out.
- Someone stayed. Presence mattered more than perfection.

- Someone helped connect to care. A counselor, hotline, or family member stepped in.

- Faith spoke truth. God's Word and Spirit brought light into the darkness.

Turning points remind us that help is real, hope is possible, and despair does not define the end of the story.

How to Tell Stories Safely

When sharing survivor stories, keep these guidelines:

- Focus on what helped, not on methods of harm.

- Highlight hope and recovery, not just pain.

- Obtain permission if telling another person's story.

- Use stories to point toward God's grace and practical resources.

▶ Reflection

- Which story in this chapter touched me the most? Why?

- Who in my life might need to hear a story of hope right now?

- What story of God's rescue could I share with others?

♥ Scripture for Hope

"Weeping may stay for the night, but rejoicing comes in the morning." (Psalm 30:5)

Reflections and Prayer

Chapter 8
– Families, Friends, and Pastors –

Suicidal crises rarely happen in isolation. When someone struggles with despair, their family, friends, and faith leaders often become the first line of support. But many loved ones feel unsure, afraid, or unprepared. What do you say? What if you make it worse? This chapter provides guidance for those who want to help but don't know how.

The Power of Presence

The most important gift is not perfect words it is presence. Families and friends often underestimate how much it means simply to stay close.

- Sit with the person.
- Listen more than you speak.
- Offer reassurance: "I'm here, and I'm not leaving."

Presence pushes back against the lie of isolation. It reminds the hurting person: "I matter enough for someone to stay."

What to Say and What Not to Say

Helpful words:

- "I'm so sorry you're hurting."
- "I want to understand what you're going through."
- "You are not alone we'll get through this together."

Unhelpful words:

- "You just need more faith."
- "Think about how this would hurt your family."
- "Other people have it worse."

The goal is not to fix the pain with words, but to validate the struggle and open the door for hope.

Boundaries for Helpers

While presence matters, helpers must also set healthy boundaries. No one person can carry the full weight of another's despair.

- Share responsibility: involve other family members, friends, or professionals.
- Avoid secrecy: if someone is in danger, tell a trusted professional or emergency services.
- Care for yourself: counseling, prayer, and rest for helpers are essential.

You cannot pour from an empty cup. Supporting someone else requires filling your own.

Pastors and Spiritual Leaders

Pastors are often the first people members of a congregation turn to in crisis. Yet many pastors feel unequipped. Churches can prepare by:

- Training leaders to recognize warning signs.
- Establishing referral networks with local counselors.
- Preaching openly about mental health, despair, and hope in Christ.
- Offering pastoral counseling alongside professional care.

A pastor's role is not to replace a doctor or therapist but to provide spiritual guidance, prayer, and connection to resources.

The Ministry of Listening

Sometimes the most pastoral act is not preaching but listening. When people feel heard without judgment, they often find strength to seek further help.

"Everyone should be quick to listen, slow to speak and slow to become angry." (James 1:19)

Listening is ministry. It validates pain and creates space for healing.

Helping Families Walk Together

Suicidal thoughts affect the entire household. Families can:

- Hold family prayer times focused on comfort and hope.
- Learn about risk factors and warning signs together.
- Create a home environment of openness and safety.
- Support one another with encouragement and grace.

Families who walk together in love often become lifelines for one another.

Survivor Story: "My Mom's Persistence"

"When I wanted to give up, my mom kept checking in. She didn't lecture — she just asked how I was really doing. Sometimes I snapped at her, but she didn't stop. Her persistence showed me I mattered. It eventually gave me the courage to get help."

Faith in Action

Faith leaders and family members can put faith into action by:

- Praying with the person, not just for them.
- Reading Scripture aloud that affirms worth and hope.
- Reminding them gently of God's promises: "Never will I leave you; never will I forsake you." (Hebrews 13:5)

Faith without compassion feels empty; faith expressed through presence brings life.

▶ Reflection

- How comfortable am I with listening without trying to "fix" right away?
- What boundaries do I need to set so I can support others without burning out?
- How can my family or church become more prepared to respond to crisis?

♥ Scripture for Hope

"Carry each other's burdens, and in this way you will fulfill the law of Christ." (Galatians 6:2)

Reflections and Prayer

Chapter 9
– The Church is a Lifeline –

The church is meant to be more than a gathering place. It is the body of Christ, called to be His hands and feet in a hurting world. For those battling suicidal thoughts, the church can either be a place of shame and silence or a refuge of hope and healing. This chapter explores how the church can step into it's role as a lifeline a safe community where despair is met with compassion and truth.

Why the Church Matters

The church is uniquely positioned to address suicide because it offers what the world cannot:

- Spiritual hope rooted in Christ's victory over death.

- Community support that surrounds people with love.

- Purpose and meaning beyond the present pain.

When the church speaks honestly about despair and models Christ's compassion, it becomes a place where lives are saved.

Breaking the Silence

Too often, suicide has been a taboo subject in churches. Avoiding the topic creates shame and isolation. Breaking the silence means:

- Preaching openly about mental health and despair.

- Using testimonies of God's redemption to encourage others.

- Including suicide prevention resources in church bulletins, websites, and sermons.

Silence communicates rejection. Openness communicates welcome.

Training Leaders to Respond

Pastors, elders, and ministry leaders must be equipped to respond when someone confides in suicidal thoughts. Training should include:

- Recognizing warning signs.
- Asking direct questions without fear.
- Connecting individuals to professional help.
- Providing spiritual care through prayer and Scripture.

Churches can partner with local counselors or host workshops to build confidence among leaders.

Creating Safe Spaces

People are more likely to seek help when they feel safe. Churches can create safe spaces by:

- Establishing confidential support groups.
- Offering pastoral counseling alongside professional referrals.
- Providing a culture of grace rather than judgment.
- Encouraging testimony, honesty, and lament in worship.

A church that welcomes honest pain mirrors Christ, who invited the weary and brokenhearted to come to Him.

The Role of Small Groups

Small groups can be lifelines within the larger church body. They provide:

- Accountability and regular check-ins.
- Opportunities for members to share struggles without fear.

- Prayer and encouragement during difficult weeks.
- A network that notices when someone withdraws.

When small groups function as families, people in despair are less likely to feel invisible.

Partnering with Professionals

The church should never attempt to replace professional mental health care. Instead, it should complement it. Practical partnerships may include:

- Hosting counseling sessions in church facilities.
- Referring members to Christian counselors or community clinics.
- Supporting members with follow-up and encouragement after counseling sessions.

Partnership demonstrates humility — acknowledging that God uses both faith and professional wisdom to bring healing.

Survivor Story: "The Church That Saved My Life"

"When I admitted to my small group that I was thinking about suicide, I expected them to push me away. Instead, they prayed with me, sat with me, and even called a counselor for me. They walked with me every step of the way. I truly believe my church family saved my life.

Theological Foundations of Hope

The church proclaims the gospel of life:

- Jesus defeated death (1 Corinthians 15:55–57).
- Nothing separates us from God's love (Romans 8:38–39).
- We are God's workmanship, created with purpose (Ephesians 2:10).

These truths anchor the church's response to suicide. Theology without compassion feels cold. Compassion without truth feels shallow. Together, they form a lifeline.

Practical Steps for Churches

- Host an annual "Hope Sunday" focused on mental health and suicide prevention.
- Train greeters, ushers, and volunteers to recognize distress.
- Provide resource tables with crisis hotline numbers.
- Encourage testimonies of God's deliverance from despair.
- Create a referral list of Christian counselors, clinics, and crisis lines.

▶ Reflection

- How has my church responded to despair in the past?
- What barriers keep my congregation from talking openly about suicide?
- What first step could we take this month to become a lifeline?

♥ Scripture for Hope

"Therefore encourage one another and build each other up, just as in fact you are doing." (1 Thessalonians 5:11)

Reflections and Prayer

Chapter 10
– After a Crisis – Healing the Soul –

When the immediate danger has passed, the work of healing begins. A suicidal crisis is not only an emergency; it is also a wound to the mind, body, and spirit. Survivors often carry lingering feelings of shame, fear, or exhaustion. Families may feel uncertain about what comes next. Churches may wonder how best to support recovery. This chapter explores the journey of restoration — how to walk with God and with others toward wholeness after the storm.

The Lingering Impact of Crisis

Surviving a suicidal moment does not mean the pain disappears overnight. Many describe feeling:

- Ashamed for having had suicidal thoughts.
- Exhausted from the intensity of the crisis.
- Afraid that the thoughts may return.
- Unsure of how to explain what happened to loved ones.

These emotions are normal. Healing begins by acknowledging them without judgment

The Gift of Grace

Shame often lingers longer than the crisis itself. Survivors may think, "If people knew what I thought, they'd see me differently." But God's Word tells a different story:

"Therefore, there is now no condemnation for those who are in Christ Jesus." (Romans 8:1)

The grace of Christ removes condemnation. In Him, our past does not define us. Healing the soul requires receiving grace both from God and from ourselves.

The Role of Counseling After Crisis

Post-crisis counseling helps survivors process what happened and build resilience. Key goals include:

- Identifying triggers that led to the crisis.
- Developing coping strategies for future stress.
- Addressing underlying issues such as trauma, grief, or abuse.
- Restoring self-worth and confidence.

For some, group therapy or support groups provide additional encouragement. Hearing "me too" from others removes isolation.

Family Healing After Crisis

Crisis affects not only the individual but also the family. Loved ones may feel guilt, fear, or confusion. Families can heal by:

- Talking openly about the crisis without blame.
- Attending family counseling or pastoral care sessions together.
- Learning how to support without smothering.
- Practicing patience recognizing that recovery takes time.

When families respond with love and grace, they become powerful partners in healing.

Pastoral Care in Recovery

Pastors and church leaders play a vital role beyond the crisis. Spiritual care may include:

- Visiting or calling regularly to check in.
- Offering prayer for peace and renewed purpose.
- Guiding the person into small groups or ministry opportunities.
- Preaching messages that normalize lament while pointing to hope.

The church becomes a healing community when it combines truth, love, and presence.

Faith Practices That Restore the Soul

Daily rhythms of faith help survivors rebuild hope:

- Prayer of lament: Honest prayers like the Psalms, naming pain before God.
- Scripture meditation: Verses on God's promises of presence and worth.
- Worship: Singing truth over feelings of despair.
- Service: Helping others rekindles purpose and dignity.

"He restores my soul. He guides me along the right paths for His name's sake." (Psalm 23:3)

Faith does not erase the crisis, but it reorients the soul toward the God who restores

Survivor Story: "Life After the Attempt"

"After my attempt, I felt like everyone would see me differently. I was embarrassed and afraid. But my church surrounded me with love. My pastor told me, 'This is not who you are. This is something you survived.' Over time, I realized God was giving me a second chance — not just to live, but to live with new purpose."

Walking Toward Purpose

Healing is not just about moving away from despair; it is about moving toward meaning. Survivors who thrive often discover:

- A renewed sense of calling.
- Opportunities to serve others with compassion.
- A testimony that encourages others still in the valley.

Purpose transforms survival into significance.

▶ Reflection

- What emotions linger after a crisis in me or in someone I love?
- How can I practice grace toward myself or others in recovery?
- What steps could help me (or someone I know) rediscover purpose?

♥ Scripture for Hope

"The Lord upholds all who fall and lifts up all who are bowed down." (Psalm 145:14

Reflections and Prayer

Chapter II
– Grief and the Aftermath –

When suicide takes a life, it leaves behind a storm of questions, emotions, and pain. Families and friends often struggle with guilt, anger, confusion, or shame. Churches may feel unsure how to respond. Grief after suicide is unlike any other it is heavy, complicated, and often isolating. Yet even here, God's comfort and healing can meet us. This chapter explores how to process grief, walk with others in sorrow, and find hope after devastating loss.

The Unique Pain of Suicide Loss

All grief is painful, but suicide loss carries unique weight:

- Unanswered questions: "Why didn't I see it? What could I have done?"
- Guilt: "If only I had called that night…"
- Anger: at the person, at circumstances, sometimes even at God.
- Stigma: fear of what others will think or say.
- Isolation: feeling alone in a grief others may not understand.

Naming this pain helps us see it for what it is: not weakness, but the human response to a heartbreaking loss.

God's Presence in Grief

The Bible assures us:

"The Lord is close to the brokenhearted and saves those who are crushed in spirit." (Psalm 34:18)

God does not shy away from our grief. He meets us in the valley, offering presence even when answers are absent. Jesus Himself wept at Lazarus's tomb (John 11:35), reminding us that tears are holy and grief is sacred.

The Weight of Guilt

Survivors of suicide loss often replay the past, searching for missed signs. This guilt can feel crushing. Yet it is important to remember: one person does not hold the power of another's choices. Suicide is complex, involving many factors. Blaming oneself only deepens the wound.

Romans 8:1 reminds us: "Therefore, there is now no condemnation for those who are in Christ Jesus." This includes those who grieve what they could not control.

Anger and Questions for God

Anger is a natural part of grief. Some feel anger at the person who died; others feel anger at God for allowing it. The Psalms give us permission to bring these raw emotions to Him:

"How long, Lord? Will you forget me forever? How long will you hide your face from me?" (Psalm 13:1)

God can handle our honest questions. He does not turn away from lament; He welcomes it

How Families Can Heal Together

Families touched by suicide can support each other by:

- Speaking openly about their grief.
- Avoiding blame or secrecy.
- Seeking counseling, individually and as a family.
- Remembering the loved one in healthy ways (memorials, stories, traditions).
- Leaning on faith practices: prayer, Scripture, worship.

Healing does not mean forgetting. It means learning to carry the memory with grace rather than despair.

The Role of the Church After Suicide

Churches often struggle with how to respond after suicide. Some avoid mentioning it, fearing they might cause pain. But silence can deepen stigma. Instead, churches can:

- Offer pastoral care visits and grief support groups.
- Acknowledge the loss openly in prayer and compassion.
- Provide safe spaces for families to share their stories.
- Offer ongoing care beyond the funeral service.

A compassionate church presence can be a vital lifeline for grieving families.

Survivor Story: "Finding Hope After Loss"

"When my brother died by suicide, I felt completely alone. I thought people would judge us. But my church surrounded us with meals, prayers, and presence. They didn't try to explain it away. They simply loved us. Over time, I realized God was still with me, even in the questions I couldn't answer."

Finding Meaning in the Aftermath

Grief does not disappear, but many survivors eventually find meaning by:

- Supporting others who face similar loss.
- Advocating for suicide prevention.
- Sharing their story as a testimony of God's sustaining grace.
- Remembering their loved one in ways that bring life, not despair.

As Paul writes:

> "Praise be to the God... who comforts us in all our troubles, so that we can comfort those in any trouble with the comfort we ourselves receive from God." (2 Corinthians 1:3–4)

▶ Reflection

- What emotions do I feel most strongly in grief, guilt, anger, sadness, or something else?
- How can I invite God into my honest questions?
- What steps can I take to remember my loved one in life-giving ways?

♥ Scripture for Hope

> "He will wipe every tear from their eyes. There will be no more death or mourning or crying or pain, for the old order of things has passed away." (Revelation 21:4)

Reflections and Prayer

Chapter 12
– Prevention at Scale –

Suicide is not only an individual struggle, it is also a public health issue and a community challenge. While personal compassion saves lives in the moment, systemic prevention can reduce risk for entire populations. This chapter explores what it means to respond at scale: in neighborhoods, schools, workplaces, churches, and nations.

Why Prevention Matters

Every year, more than 700,000 people worldwide die by suicide. For every life lost, there are countless attempts and millions of grieving family members left behind. Prevention matters because suicide is not inevitable it is preventable.

Prevention at scale creates layers of protection so that when individuals reach moments of crisis, they are more likely to find safety, support, and hope.

Public Health Approaches

Public health strategies include:

- Education and Awareness: teaching warning signs, risk factors, and how to ask about suicide.

- Means Restriction: reducing access to lethal methods (e.g., firearm safety, safe storage of medications).

- Crisis Services: expanding hotlines, text lines, and mobile crisis units.

- School Programs: teaching coping skills and resilience to young people.
- Workplace Initiatives: training employees and supervisors to recognize distress.

When these measures are put in place, communities see measurable decreases in suicide rates.

The Role of Churches in Community Prevention

Churches are not only spiritual centers, they are also community hubs. They can:

- Partner with schools to host mental health awareness nights.
- Offer facilities for support groups and counseling.
- Train volunteers to serve as crisis responders.
- Share hotline numbers and prevention resources in bulletins and online.
- Build partnerships with local hospitals and crisis centers.

When churches lead, stigma is reduced, and hope is multiplied.

Global and National Strategies

Organizations like the World Health Organization (WHO) and the Centers for Disease Control and Prevention (CDC) have identified key strategies:

- Building national suicide prevention plans.
- Expanding access to mental health services.
- Increasing funding for research and training.
- Promoting media guidelines to report suicide responsibly.

Faith communities can align with these strategies, adding the message of Christ's hope to the foundation of public health.

Faith and Prevention

Faith provides unique contributions to prevention:

- Meaning: reminding people that life has eternal worth.
- Community: offering belonging that counteracts isolation.
- Hope: declaring that despair does not have the final word.

Scripture speaks to prevention when it says:

"Rescue those being led away to death; hold back those staggering toward slaughter." (Proverbs 24:11)

This is the church's call to action.

Practical Ways Individuals Can Contribute

You don't need to be a professional to play a role in prevention. You can:

- Share the 988 Lifeline (U.S.) or local crisis numbers with your network.
- Take a training course such as QPR (Question, Persuade, Refer) or ASIST (Applied Suicide Intervention Skills Training).
- Volunteer at a crisis center or church support group.
- Advocate for policies that fund mental health care and prevention programs.
- Speak openly about your own story of survival or support.

Every act of awareness and compassion strengthens the safety net.

Survivor Story: "From Despair to Advocacy"

"After my son's suicide, I decided his life would not be forgotten. I started speaking at schools about warning signs and prevention. At first, it was hard to share. But now I see his story is saving lives. God has turned my pain into purpose."

The Ripple Effect of Prevention

When prevention is embraced at scale:

- Families are more open about struggles.
- Schools equip students with coping tools.
- Churches become safe places for confession and healing.
- Communities reduce stigma and increase support.

Each ripple contributes to fewer lives lost and more lives transformed.

▶ Reflection

- What prevention strategies could my church or community implement this year?
- How can I personally contribute to reducing stigma and spreading hope?
- What step can I take to align faith with prevention in my own circle of influence?

♥ Scripture for Hope

"You are the light of the world. A town built on a hill cannot be hidden." (Matthew 5:14)

Reflections and Prayer

Conclusion
– Life Beyond the Moment –

This book began with a conviction: suicide is a moment of thought, not a mental illness. Along the way, we have explored the science of crisis, the role of faith, the importance of families and churches, and the ways prevention can happen on a scale. Now we come to the heart of the matter: what does it mean to live beyond the moment?

The Thought Is Not the End

Suicidal thoughts are real. They are heavy, frightening, and overwhelming. But they are not final. They are not identity. They are not destiny. They are a moment and moments pass.

When the storm of despair rages, it may feel like the end of the story. But God reminds us that He is still writing:

"For I know the plans I have for you," declares the Lord, "plans to prosper you and not to harm you, plans to give you hope and a future." (Jeremiah 29:11

Choosing Life Daily

Living beyond the moment means choosing life again and again sometimes daily, sometimes minute by minute. It is not about never feeling despair again; it is about remembering that despair does not define the future.

Choosing life may look like:

- Reaching out for help instead of staying silent.
- Practicing faith disciplines like prayer, worship, and Scripture reading.
- Building community through church, friendships, and small groups.
- Seeking professional care when needed.
- Serving others to rediscover meaning and purpose.

Every small choice builds strength for tomorrow.

From Survival to Significance

Survival is the first step; significance is the next. God does not only want us to survive He wants us to thrive and live with purpose. Many who once faced suicidal thoughts later find deep joy in helping others through their own storms.

Paul wrote:

"Praise be to the God… who comforts us in all our troubles, so that we can comfort those in any trouble with the comfort we ourselves receive from God." (2 Corinthians 1:3–4)

Your pain can become someone else's lifeline. Your survival can become someone else's testimony of hope.

The Church's Call to Action

The body of Christ is called to be a refuge for the broken, a hospital for the hurting, and a lighthouse for the lost. Suicide prevention is not separate from the gospel it is the gospel in action. It is rescuing those led away to death (Proverbs 24:11). It is loving people as Christ loved us (John 13:34).

Every church has the opportunity to be a place where people confess despair and find compassion, where shame is replaced with grace, and where hopelessness is met with the living hope of Christ.

A Final Word of Hope

If you are reading these words and struggling with thoughts of suicide, know this: you are not alone. Your life is precious. Your story is not finished. This moment of thought does not define you.

Call out to God He is near. Reach out to someone, a teacher a friend, a pastor they care. Take one more step, one more breath, one more moment. There is life beyond this thought, and there is hope beyond this moment.

"I have come that they may have life, and have it to the full." (John 10:10)

▶ Reflection

- What is one truth I want to carry with me from this book?
- Who in my life could I encourage with hope today?
- How can I live each day with renewed purpose and meaning in Christ?

♥ Scripture for Hope

"For you created my inmost being; you knit me together in my mother's womb. I praise you because I am fearfully and wonderfully made." (Psalm 139:13–14)

Reflections and Prayer

Letters of Hope and Healing
– God is Still Holding Your Hand –

Real Stories, Real Hope Edition

"For I am the Lord your God who takes hold of your right hand and says to you, Do not fear; I will help you." — Isaiah 41:13

Before you begin, breathe... BREATHE again... And BREATHE deeper to feel the presence of God holding your right hand.

It's okay to not be okay. It's not okay to harm yourself when there is help here for you. If you are struggling, call or text 988 — the Suicide & Crisis Lifeline. You are not alone.

According to national statistics, suicide remains one of the leading causes of death in the United States — especially among young people. Every day, families, schools, churches, and communities quietly lose someone they love. It is estimated that one in five high school students has seriously considered suicide, and suicide among those ages 10–24 has increased over 60% since 2007. Adults and seniors are not untouched; loneliness, loss, and hidden depression weigh heavily across generations.

These numbers are not cold data, they are faces, families, and stories. They are people who were laughing yesterday and cried alone last night. The truth is simple: this is really happening. But so is hope. Hope is happening right now through those who choose to stay, to reach out, to breathe one more breath and whisper, "God, please help me."

These letters are written for them, for you and for every heart still beating in the middle of the storm.

Letter 1: To the One Who Feels Unseen

STOP. You are not invisible; you are exhausted.

J.L., 16 (Student): She turned in her homework early, stayed quiet in class, and walked home with her earbuds in. No one texted. No one asked. She smiled at dinner, but her heart whispered, "Does anyone see me?"
R.M., 42 (Mother): She cleaned, worked, paid bills, answered questions, but no one said, "Thank you." Only, "Can you do more?" She sighed, "I can't keep this up," then folded one more load of laundry.

Dear Self:
Today I felt invisible. I did so much, and it felt like no one noticed. I keep saying yes because I want peace, but I'm losing mine. It's okay to say no. God is not asking me to carry the world only to walk with Him. I matter, even when I feel unseen. Lord, help me ask, "What do You need of me?"

God's Whisper:
"My child, I see you when no one else does. You are not invisible to Me. You are loved — fully, always."

Pause · Pray · Plan
- Pause: Breathe. Feel your heartbeat it's proof that God's still working.
- Pray: "Lord, remind me that my worth isn't measured by what I do."
- Plan: Say this once today: "Not right now. I need to rest."

Let's pray this together:
"God, for everyone who feels unseen tonight, open our eyes to each other. Let someone's glance, text, or smile remind them: they are known and loved."

"The Lord is close to the brokenhearted." Psalm 34:18

Letter 2: To the One Who Feels Like a Burden

STOP. That voice saying "You're too much" is lying.

A.C., 19 (College Student): He sat in his dorm room, scrolling past photos of friends smiling. He'd canceled plans again didn't want to "drag anyone down." He whispered, "They'd be better off without me." God whispered louder, "No, they wouldn't."

Dear Self:
I'm tired of needing help. But I am not a burden. My weakness doesn't make me unworthy — it's where grace begins. I don't have to apologize for existing. I am not too much for the God who carried the cross.

God's Whisper:
"You are not a problem to solve. You are a person to love."

Pause · Pray · Plan
- Pause: Identify one lie — and name it false.
- Pray: "Lord, show me someone safe I can reach out to."
- Plan: Text one person: "Could we talk? I need someone today."

Let's pray this together:
"God, be near those who feel they're in the way. Show them they matter. Let them see that needing help is not failure it's faith."

"Cast all your anxiety on Him because He cares for you." 1 Peter 5:7

Letter 3: To the One Whose Pain Won't Stop

STOP. Pain is not the end it's a signal it's time to know who you are with God.

K.D., 28 (Teacher): She smiled in class but cried in the car. She thought, "If one more thing goes wrong, I can't handle it." Yet that night, she opened her Bible to Psalm 147: "He heals the brokenhearted." She stayed.

Dear Self:
The ache feels endless, but I'm still here. I don't have to hide pain from God. He's not ashamed of me. My story doesn't end in pain it begins again in healing.

God's Whisper:
"You are allowed to hurt and still hope. I am not disappointed in your weakness."

Pause · Pray · Plan
- Pause: Feel the ground beneath your feet you are still standing.
- Pray: "Lord, turn my pain into purpose."
- Plan: Tell someone, "Today is hard, but I'm still here."

Let's pray this together:
"God, hold every person fighting unseen battles tonight. Give them one reason to keep breathing — Your presence."

"He heals the brokenhearted and binds up their wounds." Psalm 147:3

Letter 4: To the One Grieving a Suicide Loss

STOP. You could not have saved them alone.

S.W., 54 (Father): He stares at a photo on the mantel, replaying "what if" on loop. The guilt is heavy, but God never asked him to be a savior only a father.

Dear Self:
I keep replaying the past, wondering what I missed. But love didn't fail. I didn't fail. Grief is not guilt. I can honor their life by living mine.

God's Whisper:
"You did what you could. I am holding them and you."

Pause · Pray · Plan
- Pause: Speak their name aloud. Love still reaches heaven.
- Pray: "Jesus, help me forgive what I couldn't control."
- Plan: Share one story of their life with someone new.

Let's pray this together:
"God, comfort those who mourn tonight. Remind us that love never dies in You."

"Blessed are those who mourn, for they will be comforted."
Matthew 5:4

Letter 5: To the One Ready to Give Up

STOP. This is not you're ending.

M.R., 23 (Veteran): He sat in silence, phone in hand, scrolling through numbers but calling none. He thought, "I don't want to die. I just don't want to hurt." God whispered, "Then let Me help you heal."

According to national data, someone attempts suicide every 40 seconds but just as often, someone chooses to stay. You can be that someone.

Dear Self:
I am exhausted. I can't see the way forward. But God, if You're still here, show me how to stay. Even if I take just one breath at a time, help me believe you still have purpose for me.

God's Whisper:
"This is not you're ending. I am still writing your story."

Pause · Pray · Plan
- Pause: Say your name — it still matters.
- Pray: "Jesus, interrupt me with peace."
- Plan: Call or text 988 right now. Let someone walk you through this night.

Let's pray this together:
"God, for every heart ready to give up, surround them with Your presence. Show them one reason to live tonight."

"The Lord will fight for you; you need only to be still." — Exodus 14:14

Letter 6: To the One Being Strong for Everyone

STOP. You don't have to hold everyone up.

L.N., 37 (Pastor): He preaches hope every Sunday but collapses in silence on Monday. He whispers, "I can't keep saving everyone else." God answers, "You're not their Savior, I am."

Dear Self:
I keep carrying what isn't mine. But I can't pour from an empty cup. It's holy to rest. It's faithful to say, "I can't." Lord, teach me to rest in You.

God's Whisper:
"My child, it's not weakness to need Me. It's wisdom."

Pause · Pray · Plan
- Pause: Set down what's not yours to carry.
- Pray: "Lord, help me release what I can't control."
- Plan: Schedule rest as worship. Say, "No," and mean it.

Let's pray this together:
"God, give courage to the strong ones who secretly struggle. Let them feel safe to fall into Your arms."

"Be still and know that I am God." — Psalm 46:10

Letter 7: To the One Ready to Begin Again

STOP. Look: morning came again.

T.D., 72 (Widower): He sat by the window, coffee trembling in his hands. The ache of loss still heavy, yet a bird sang on the sill. He smiled through tears and whispered, "Thank You, Lord."

Dear Self:
Today isn't perfect, but it's new. I can forgive what I couldn't change. I am not who pain said I was. I am who God says I am — His.

God's Whisper:
"Behold, I make all things new."

Pause · Pray · Plan
- Pause: Thank God for one small mercy you see.
- Pray: "Lord, guide me one step at a time."
- Plan: Write a short list: (1) Connect with God, (2) Care for my body, (3) Reach someone who needs me.

Let's pray this together:
"God, thank You for new beginnings. Help us believe that the sunrise means You're not done."

"For I know the plans I have for you… plans to give you hope and a future." — Jeremiah 29:11

Truth to Hold On To

You are not alone.
This pain is not the end of your story.
Right now, countless others are fighting the same fight
— and God is holding every hand at once.

If You Are in Crisis

If you are in emotional pain or thinking of self-harm,
please reach out now.
Call or text **988** to connect with the Suicide & Crisis Lifeline
— available 24/7.
You are not alone. God is with you. We are with you.

Appendix A: Personal Safety Plan

(Use this section as a fillable or reflective guide for moments of crisis.)

"The Lord is my strength and my shield; my heart trusts in Him, and He helps me." — *Psalm 28:7*

When despair feels overwhelming, a plan can save your life. This personal safety plan is meant to guide you step-by-step toward safety, faith, and support.

1. Warning Signs That I Might Be in Crisis

These are thoughts, feelings, or behaviors that tell me I'm struggling:

2. Internal Coping Strategies

Things I can do to calm myself without calling anyone:

3. People and Places That Help Me Feel Safe

- Safe spaces (church, park, favorite room): _____

- People I can spend time with safely: _____

4. Who I Can Call for Help

- Friend: _____
- Family member: _____
- Pastor or mentor: _____

5. Professional or Crisis Contacts

- My counselor or therapist: _____
- Doctor: _____
- **Suicide & Crisis Lifeline (U.S.): Dial or Text 988**
- **If outside the U.S.:** Visit *findahelpline.com* for local numbers.

6. Steps to Make My Environment Safer

- Remove or secure harmful items.
- Store medications safely.
- Ask someone to hold onto anything that could be used for harm.

7. My Reasons for Living and God's Promises

- What reminds me that my life still has purpose: _____
- Scriptures that bring me peace: _____

"He heals the brokenhearted and binds up their wounds." — *Psalm 147:3*

Appendix B: Conversation Scripts

(For helpers, friends, and pastors)

"Everyone should be quick to listen, slow to speak..." — *James 1:19*

When someone confides that they are thinking about suicide, your response matters more than perfect words. Use these simple, compassionate approaches.

1. How to Ask Directly

- "Are you thinking about suicide?"
- "Sometimes when people feel hopeless, they think about ending their life. Are you thinking that way?"

2. When They Say Yes

- "Thank you for trusting me. I'm really glad you told me."
- "You are not alone. I want to help you stay safe tonight."
- "Let's call or text 988 together, or I can stay with you while we get help."

3. When You Must Call for Help

If someone is in danger, call 911 (U.S.) or your local emergency number immediately. Stay calm and remain with them until help arrives.

4. Faith-Filled Encouragement

- "You are loved, even when you can't feel it."
- "God's not angry — He's reaching out to you right now."
- "I'll pray with you, but I'll also walk with you."

5. Follow-Up

- Check in the next day: "How are you doing today? I'm still here."
- Encourage professional and faith-based care.
- Never assume the crisis is over after one conversation.

"The Lord will fight for you; you need only to be still."
— *Exodus 14:14*

Appendix C: Scriptures of Hope

"The entrance of Your words gives light." — *Psalm 119:130*

Use these verses as daily anchors when despair whispers lies.

Isaiah 41:10 — "So do not fear, for I am with you."
Psalm 34:18 — "The Lord is close to the brokenhearted."
Romans 8:38–39 — "Nothing can separate us from the love of God."
Psalm 23:4 — "Even though I walk through the darkest valley, You are with me."
2 Corinthians 1:3–4 — "The God of all comfort… comforts us in all our troubles."
Jeremiah 29:11 — "Plans to give you hope and a future."
Psalm 147:3 — "He heals the brokenhearted."
Philippians 4:7 — "The peace of God… will guard your hearts and your minds."
John 10:10 — "I have come that they may have life, and have it to the full."
1 Peter 1:3 — "A living hope through the resurrection of Jesus Christ."
Matthew 11:28 — "Come to Me, all you who are weary and burdened."
Psalm 139:14 — "I praise You because I am fearfully and wonderfully made."
Hebrews 13:5 — "Never will I leave you; never will I forsake you."
Revelation 21:4 — "He will wipe every tear from their eyes."

Appendix D: Resources & Crisis Guide

Immediate Help (United States)

988 Suicide & Crisis Lifeline
– Call or text **988** (24/7, confidential, free)
– Chat online: 988lifeline.org

Veterans Crisis Line
– Call **988**, then press **1**
– Text 838255

Crisis Text Line
– Text **HOME** to **741741**

International Help

Visit findahelpline.com for hotlines in over 100 countries. Examples:

- **UK:** Samaritans — 116 123
- **Canada:** Talk Suicide Canada — 1-833-456-4566
- **Australia:** Lifeline — 13 11 14

Faith-Based and Counseling Resources

- **Focus on the Family Counseling Service:** 1-855-771-HELP (4357)
- **American Association of Christian Counselors:** www.aacc.net
- **Celebrate Recovery:** www.celebraterecovery.com
- **National Alliance on Mental Illness (NAMI) HelpLine:** 1-800-950-NAMI (6264)

Local & Ministry Contact

Rapha Christian Counseling Center & Academic Institute
www.raphaccc.org
info@raphaccc.org

"Rescue those being led away to death; hold back those staggering toward slaughter." — *Proverbs 24:11*

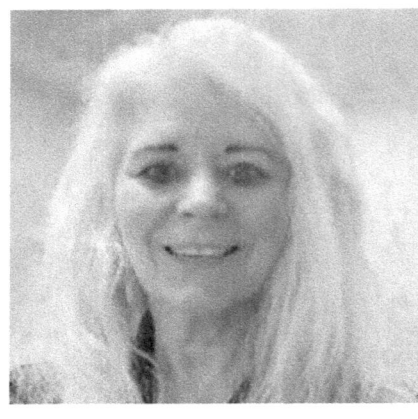

About the Author

Dr. Janet Olivares, founder and CEO of **Rapha Christian Counseling Center & Academic Institute**, is a counselor, teacher, wife, mother, grandmother, and great-grandmother whose life's work is devoted to restoring hope and emotional healing through Christ-centered care. Her leadership has guided countless individuals and families toward renewed peace and purpose through professional Christian counseling and education.

Her counseling philosophy is rooted in grace — believing that no one is beyond God's ability to heal, and that faith and mental health can walk hand in hand.

Author's Note

There was a season in my own life when darkness whispered louder than hope. I know what it feels like to stand at the edge of despair and believe the lie that there is no way forward. But I also know the miracle of God's mercy — how He steps into the quiet, takes hold of our right hand, and says, *"Do not fear; I will help you."* (Isaiah 41:13)

I share this not as confession, but as testimony. I am living proof that God restores. My story is not about what almost ended; it is about what began again when I let Him heal the parts I thought were beyond repair.

If you are walking through that valley today, know this: you are not alone. The same God who rescued me will rescue you. There is hope beyond the moment, and your story — like mine — is still being written by His hand.

— Dr. Janet Olivares

Be Sure to Check out my Other Titles:

Finding Self with God Day by Day
Forgive Let go for Real
Parental Care
Suicide: Hope Beyond a Moment
Love Never Left: Marriage Restoration

How to contact the author:
drjanet@raphaccc.org

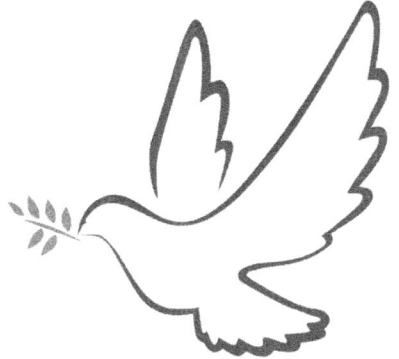

www.ingramcontent.com/pod-product-compliance
Lightning Source LLC
Chambersburg PA
CBHW070155080526
44586CB00015B/2002